Intermittent Fasting: Live Longer, Lose Weight, and Feel Great

By Katy White

I0421540

© 2015

Intermittent Fasting: Live Longer, Lose Weight, and Feel Great

Are you tired of trying a different diet every month? Have you tried eating small meals throughout the day, or maybe 3 big meals per day? Have you cut carbs, cut fat, cut sugar, and more? Are you still not meeting your healthy living and weight-loss goals?

With Intermittent Fasting, you can say goodbye to all of these problems and say hello to the healthy life and body you've always wanted!

In this book, you'll find out what intermittent fasting is, how it works, what benefits you can expect, and how to get started right away! All the different methods of intermittent fasting are included so you can easily try out different methods and select the one that suits your lifestyle best.

This book is your complete guide to Intermittent Fasting. You can get started right away and jump-start your healthy lifestyle and weight loss journey today!

Intermittent Fasting

It is the new craze in dieting. And it's not even really dieting. It is called Intermittent Fasting. Have you heard of it? It basically means you fast for an extended period of time. Say you fast through your sleep, which you do already, if you do not eat in your sleep. Now, if you extend the time until you eat for a few more hours, you are Intermittent Fasting. Intermittent Fasting means to be more conscious of your fasting and feeding schedule. It really is not as hard as it sounds, and the results can be incredible!

Is dieting hard? Yes, there is no doubt about it. It is extremely hard to worry about eating too much each and every day. I constantly worry about what I am going to have for dinner the next day and pray that I do not end up in bed starving! Now that is a nightmare. Plus, you are riddled with guilt when you eat something with as many carbs as a bagel. It haunts you sometimes, does it not? Or maybe there is a day when someone brings donuts to the office and you just need to have one because you have not eaten anything delicious in weeks. Do not worry. This is not a problem with Intermittent Fasting! Dieting can be easy!

No, I am not kidding. Dieting can be easy. Look, I said it again. How? Let me tell you about Intermittent Fasting. You may have heard of people fasting when they give something up for a period of time or refrain from eating within a certain window, like during

Ramadan or Lent. It is essentially the same idea. Intermittent Fasting is about refraining from eating during a specific time frame.

Wait! It is actually much easier than it sounds. Essentially, we all fast when we sleep. Unless you have a habit of sleep walking to the fridge and then eating in your sleep, you generally fast during your sleep. That is why the first meal of the day is called "breakfast" because you are breaking your fast. If you sleep 8 hours, you will most likely have fasted at least 8 hours, if not more, depending on when you eat your last meal and when you eat your first meal. That does not sound so bad, now, does it?

For years we have been pounded with the idea that we need to eat at certain times, and if we miss that window, our metabolism will go down. Well, recent studies have proven that to be completely incorrect. The only true and accepted rule of dieting is that the calories in have to be less than calories out. That is how you lose weight, period. There are no magic methods. This is your equation. The amount of calories that you consume has to be less than you use up! It is a simple enough math problem, but sometimes, you can make this equation easier.

Intermittent Fasting is one of those ways.

If you feel skeptical about Intermittent Fasting because scientists have jammed into our brains the need to eat consistently throughout the day, then note this: cavemen would fast during periods of times when food was scarce. Yes, just like the paleo diet, Intermittent Fasting has roots in our caveman history. Perhaps we have been spoiled by our ability to access food on a regular basis or maybe it is the fact that scientists have scared us with tales of metabolic damage. Wherever the fear comes from, we need to understand that it is perfectly fine for us to consume low levels of calories for a prolonged period of time. Not only is it fine, it can be downright healthy!

I think it is most definitely time to stop accepting theories as truth and explore what truly works in our own lives! Your metabolism will not be destroyed because you wait a few hours to eat. You do not have to eat every 3 hours. Eating after 7 o'clock at night will not make you gain weight. Carbohydrates do not make you gain weight!

Wait! Do not run! I am being serious here. All of the "rules" of weight loss that you have been told for years do not need to be followed anymore. Why should you follow these rules? Forget them. Make dieting easier with Intermittent Fasting. Intermittent Fasting is not about rules. Intermittent Fasting is just about structure, and it helps to make your life just a bit easier. Trade in all of the rules that have ruled over you!

Now, let us get down to the nitty gritty! There are a few ways to do Intermittent Fasting, but first, let us look at the benefits versus the negatives!

Positive Effects

There have been studies done on the effects of Intermittent Fasting. One positive aspect of practicing Intermittent Fasting seems to be a heightened insulin sensitivity, which can later prove to be quite useful in combating diabetes and maintaining a healthy weight. Other benefits may include detoxification of the liver, higher growth hormone levels, and decreased inflammation depending on your preferred method of Intermittent Fasting.

For those who practice Intermittent Fasting, they may find themselves eating significantly less during their eating window. For those who desire to gain muscle, they may find consuming massive amounts of food more difficult so the amount of fat gained during their bulking phase is decreased because they are not eating massive amounts of food to gain as much muscle as possible. This results in lean muscle gain. Don't worry, we'll explain this more later.

As long as you consume more than the amount of calories you need, you can build muscle, but if it is hard to eat a certain amount, you will definitely not be gaining as much fat as you usually would if you were to consume a large amount of food variously throughout the day. There are a lot of people who "bulk" by eating massive amounts of food. Guess what that means. Lots of fat gain! Intermittent Fasting can help limit that massive amount of fat gain for those who are going through their bulking phase. Intermittent Fasting has so much use for everyone!

You can also look forward to increased cellular repair and growth, blood sugar control, and fat burning. That sounds great, right? Intermittent fasting has all sorts of benefits to look forward to. However, what are the negatives? Let us find out together!

Negative Effects

The negative effects of Intermittent Fasting generally depend on the individual because everyone's body responds a little differently. For example, I would not recommend Intermittent Fasting for anyone who suffers from acid reflux. You need to eat in the morning so that you do not end up in pain the entire day. Why would I ask you to torture yourself? I wouldn't, of course. However, not everyone has acid reflux, of course, so you see, everyone has a different set of circumstances.

Now, keep in mind that you know your body the best. If you feel something changing in your mental or physical state, stop. Do you feel fine? Keep going. Do not endanger yourself. I hope I did not scare you away, but I want to make sure I thoroughly warned you first. Your health is the most important! All right, let us see what the negatives are.

One negative aspect for some is a decrease in blood pressure. When you first wake up in the morning, your blood pressure is at its lowest. It tends to spike when you eat your first meal.

Some people may find themselves light headed or unsteady if their blood pressure is too low.

That is not good for optimal performance in your training or in your work. Low blood pressure can also attribute to bad moods or mood swings. Not everyone experiences this when they skip breakfast, but it is a potential side effect for some people.

The biggest negative aspect of Intermittent Fasting to keep in mind is the transition into Intermittent Fasting. It is not an easy one because we are so attuned to eating according to eating windows and sometimes, we just think about food.

If you are not used to Intermittent Fasting, you may find your stomach growling a lot or you may be light headed at first. Take it slowly. Do not just dive into a fast. You may torture yourself that way. Maybe wait an hour after you wake up to eat the first day. Then two hours the next day. Then three, and so on and so forth. It gets easier. A lot of people who practice Intermittent Fasting find it easier to consume caffeine. It helps to suppress appetite, stop your stomach from growling, and give you energy!

The Positives and The Negatives for Me

Taking into account that I do practice Intermittent Fasting, I feel there are a great amount of benefits that I have experienced. I have been utilizing Intermittent Fasting as my main way of making my diet more flexible for over 3 years now. It has made dieting a lot easier, even when I lose control of myself and binge eat or am forced to go to buffets, high calorie dinners, and eat on the go due to a busy schedule.

While I cannot possibly notice benefits like increased cellular repair, I have noticed that my appetite has decreased exponentially and I do not feel the need to overeat. I have even seen some lean muscle gain, especially now that I am eating according to my moods instead of counting calories to an obsessive degree. I really like Intermittent Fasting now that I am doing intuitive eating because I do not worry as much about how much I am taking into my body through food. I know how to limit my consumption, but I also know that I can eat what I want should I desire to.

Also, I tend to train in a fasted state and do not usually break my fast until after 3-6 hours after training depending on the day and the condition I am in that morning, but I have not seen any significant loss in strength and I am still quite capable of performing HIIT workouts (high intensity interval training) at the end of my training sessions as well. That is pretty nice, is it not?

I think an added benefit that I had not been expecting was that my water intake increased significantly. I find I have consumed about a gallon of water before the morning is even over. Water intake is important for flushing out your system of toxins and it is good for your skin. Also, increasing your water intake is good for reducing bloating, which is a problem a lot of women have, so I was definitely happy that I bloat less. What a great, unexpected bonus!

That being said, my experience has not been all sunshine and daisies. Some days, I can tell that I have low blood pressure and lethargy. Usually, it is not a big problem unless I find my fasting window is extended more than usual or I have been awake earlier than usual. On these days, I may consume caffeine moderately throughout the day or I break my fast earlier. I find it is easier to break my fast earlier on some days if I experience any issues. Sometimes, I feel light headed so I am not going to deprive myself if my body says not to. I need treat my body with the respect it deserves, right?

When I first transitioned into Intermittent Fasting, I went from eating right when I woke up or downing a protein shake after coming back from the gym straight to a 16 hour fast starting at 9 PM and ending at 1 PM. That is not fun when you are first starting out and usually wake up at 5 in the morning to get a good workout in. That is about 8 hours after I wake until I can break my fast. Does that sound like fun to you? I had not realized there was a different window that women should take for health reasons.

Whoops! After a couple weeks, I found out I should have been doing a 14 hour window, but by that time, I was quite used to fasting for 16 hours. I have never behaved according to my gender, I suppose, so it is definitely not a surprise in the end.

I have changed my fasting times since I first started. I now start my fast at 8 PM so that I can break it a little earlier, but most days, when I busy with my work, I break my fast at around 2 PM just because I do not eat lunch until then. Somehow, without meaning to, my fasting window has gotten longer. Whoops again!

If I feel faint or lightheaded, I will break my fast early, but if I am busy, time flies. I have gone from Lean Gains to in between Lean Gains and the Warrior Diet. It may not be the ideal way of fasting, but it works for me. As long as my body continues to work well, who am I harming?

We are not the same person, so please, do not assume your body will work the same way as mine. It takes a lot of trial and error, as well as experimenting with your body and fasting times. You can go by the rules, but how many of us follow all of the rules? I know I do not!

It is very important to not be obsessive about when to end your fasting window. Yes, discipline and consistency is nice, but sometimes, your body will tell you what it wants and you should listen. Do not watch the clock madly awaiting your fasting window to end. Torturing yourself only makes it worse. If you cannot wait, then don't. Do not wait for the exact minute when your fasting window is over. That is way too obsessive. If you are starving and nothing gets rid of your hunger, then by all means, eat! Why wait an extra 10 minutes?

Intermittent Fasting and Flexible Dieting

Now, I have not explained how Intermittent Fasting works with dieting. It essentially allows you to be more flexible with your diet. The basic formula for weight loss is calories in have to be less than calories out. That means you have to burn more than you eat. That is not to say you have to start tracking the calories you eat. That can be terribly tedious. Instead, you just eat like normal.

Break your fast at lunch? Just eat lunch and then dinner. You can even have a snack if you would like. But the real benefit of intermittent fasting is you can actually eat something that may be higher in calories, if you want, and still be in a deficit.

Want that donut? You fasted, so even if you eat it, you still have a deficit. Does that burger look good? You are still in a deficit, so go for it! That does not mean you should fill your body with junk foods, of course. It means you are given the option of eating something that you may want without having to feel guilty. It's not a rigid diet prison, full of rules and off-limits foods. That's no way to live life!

Guilt is the main emotion you feel during dieting. You had a piece of bread and suddenly the world is ending. You wanted ice cream tonight so you had it, but then you feel guilty about it. All of your hard work is down the drain just because you indulged a little. It can really eat you up inside because if you had not eaten it, you would be on track, but why spend your life miserable just because you like sweets? Why kick yourself for liking certain foods.

Here is some food for thought: eating fats do not make you fat. Carbs do not make you fat. Too many calories make you fat. So stop depriving yourself of a treat when you deserve it. It is tiring to always be policing yourself and denying yourself, is it not? Why diet if you cannot enjoy life anymore? Why look like a stick if you hate every minute of your life? That is such a waste. Enjoy yourself a little. A lot! Just do not forget what truly matters in your life.

Now that I have your interest piqued, you may be wondering how people tend to fast. There are generally 5 main methods of Intermittent Fasting. Each one is different, but the concept is basically the same. You end up in a deficit either way. So let's jump in and explore them a bit more.

Lean Gains

The most common method is the Lean Gains approach, which is also known as the 16/8 rule. Did I already lose you? Do not worry, it is not really math. The 16/8 rule refers to fasting for 16 hours so you will only have an 8 hour eating window. There is only 24 hours in a day! OK, maybe I lied. There is a little math involved, but it is simple math! You will not be using too much energy to calculate those numbers.

The Lean Gains method, which was started by Martain Berhan, is the type of Intermittent Fasting you can do daily. With the Lean Gains method, you can choose what 16 hours you fast for. You can count the 8 hours that you will be sleeping for and then add another 8 hours. Maybe choose 4 hours before bed and 4 hours after waking up. Or perhaps you can start fasting 2 hours before you go to bed, and then fast for 6 hours upon waking up.

Typically, I use this method of fasting on most days. I start my fast at 8 PM and then I can end my fast at around 12 PM the next day. It is not so bad since I wake up at 6 AM to workout and will tend to eat lunch sometime after 12 PM.

Of course, there is a common acceptance that women do not have to push themselves as much because they may suffer more than men might so an acceptable fasting window for women is around 14 hours. I only use this 14 hour window if I feel some sort of side effect from fasting like dizziness but it does not affect me strongly enough to break fast sooner.

One great aspect of using the Lean Gains approach is you generally do not feel hungry during the fasting window. If you start a few hours before bed, then you barely feel the effects until a few hours after waking up.

If you train fasted, as well, you will not even notice a hungry until it is time for you to break fast, but an 8-hour feeding window is not long enough for you to feel hungry between meals. Your meals can be slightly larger, if you need, with less of a chance of overeating. Isn't that great?

Warrior Diet

The next approach would be the Warrior Diet, which was started by Ori Hofmeklr. That sounds fairly intense, does it not? I thought it sounded cool. It is similar to the Lean Gains approach but the fasting window is longer at about 20 hours while the feeding window is reduced to 4 hours. If you can stomach waiting this long, that is great! I practice this on some days when work can be busy or I am in no mood to eat in the afternoon. Once you are used to the Lean Gains approach, this can be easier to pursue on your busiest days.

However, if you decide that you want to bulk, you may find it extremely difficult to consume enough food during the 4-hour window. You might have to stuff yourself until you burst! Ouch, right? It definitely takes a warrior to pull off this diet.

I do not suggest this diet if you intend to fast 20 hours and then consume as few calories as possible on a daily basis. That is unsafe. Your body needs a certain amount of calories to function and if you are not properly consuming a certain amount, your body will not function properly and you will find your body going into starvation mode so do not even think about it! Use the warrior diet only if you intend on consuming at least your minimum needed intake. No less! I do not advocate a 500-calorie daily diet!

I think if you were disciplined enough to keep your fasting windows but undisciplined enough to prevent yourself from binge eating during your feeding window, this may be the best option. If you can stop eating for your fasting window, you can prevent yourself from over consuming because you only have 4 hours available to eat! It is a form of disciple in a way. I like structure, but I can also have issues with strictness so sometimes, it works. Do you understand what I am getting at?

Eat Stop Eat

Another alternative would be the Eat-Stop-Eat diet. It sounds simple, but the practice is a bit more difficult to handle. With the eat-stop-eat method, you are allowed to eat as you need one day and then the next day, you fast for 24 hours, and then eat normally the next day.

The idea is to create a huge deficit by not consuming a day's worth of calories. Some people may extend this fast to be 36 hours long while some may even attempt to make this 8 hours long. Yeah, if you can handle that, go for it, but the majority of the populace just fast every few days. In a 7 day week, they may have up to 2 fasting days. I think that is sufficient, do you not agree?

The eat-stop-eat method is the method promoted by Brad Pilon. The idea behind the eat-stop-eat diet is that you count your weekly calories instead of your daily calorie intake. This is how many bodybuilders and athletes work. On your strenuous exercise days, you consume more.

Then on your rest days, you decrease your intake significantly. Or in this case, you consume nothing on your rest days. It is highly inadvisable to actually train when you are not taking any food into your body. That could cause injury!

Anyway, using this method, you are roughly creating a deficit of about 2,000 to 4,000 calories depending on how many fasting days you choose to have in a week and what your feeding days are like. If you eat properly on your feeding days, you will lose weight. Also, do not think that just because you do not eat for 24 hours means you do not get to eat for a day.

If you start your fast at say 6 PM one day that means you can consume something after 6 PM the next day. That means you do not go to bed hungry! Of course, do not break your fast with some calorie laden meal or else your fast will do you no good except to prevent weight gain. I think that sounds like a lot of torture to maintain your weight, don't you think so?

A common way of doing the eat-stop-eat method of Intermittent Fasting is to combine it with the Lean Gains approach. Using this combination, you can practice Lean Gains throughout the week and then use the eat-stop-eat method 1 or 2 times during the week. Tailor the schedule to your preferences.

One variation of the eat-stop-eat diet is the 5:2 method. It basically means you have 5 normal days of eating with 2 days where you consume less than 500-600 calories depending on your gender. Of course, because women need fewer calories to function properly, women should eat on the lower side of the spectrum. Men may consume a little more because they require more for their bodies to function.

While my own experience with the eat-stop-eat method has varied, I find doing it consistently is easier than when you do it for the first time. My first 2 24-hour fasts left me lethargic, tired, and hazy, but in the later weeks, I began to get used to it and if I kept busy, I never really noticed the need to eat.

I went from doing only 1 24-hour fast to 2 24-hour fasts a week, so yes, I gradually graduated to the 5:2 diet on days when I knew I would be busy and I knew I would probably not exercise. Of course, I do not practice the eat-stop-eat method on a regular basis anymore, but sometimes, I accidentally find myself utilizing it. Hey, sometimes you are just too busy, right?

Alternate Day Diet

If you think you are too hardcore for the eat-stop-eat method, try the alternate day diet, which is the approach that was started by Dr. James Johnson and was once promoted by Dr. Krista Varady. The alternate day diet entails, as its name suggests, fasting every other day. That is not to say that you do not eat every other day because that sounds just awful. Imagine all the foods you miss out on in your life!

No, the alternate day diet means you eat normally every other day and on your fasting days, you consume at most, 500 calories. You may choose to spread your calories out throughout the day if you think you will not be able to survive not eating until evening, but most people who practice the alternate day diet find it easier to just consume 1 meal on their fasting days than attempting to stretch their calories thinly throughout the day.

OK, I am not going to lie - this sounds hard. When I was still learning about how my body worked, I gave myself 2 fasting days where I consumed only 500 calories during both days. It was easy for me to allot myself an extra piece of chocolate or a piece of cake because I felt I had earned it. Then, it went wild.

When I gained more control of myself, I was able to suppress the part of me that said I could fit in something, but those days were few.

I could never guarantee that my fasting days would go as I intended them to.

That is not to say it will not be a method that works for you, but I know myself and I know that I tend to make excuses for myself so that I can have something extra just because I worked out hard or because I am low on calories for the day. My mind likes to create the illusion that because I am on such a high deficit, I am thoroughly starved so I need more.

Then, it worsens and soon I find myself in a river of candy wrappers. Double whoops. If you are extremely disciplined, this method may work for you, but apparently my will power is lacking.

The Fat Loss Forever approach was founded by John Romaniello and Dan Go. This approach uses certain fasting aspects of the Warrior Diet, Eat-Stop-Eat approach, and Lean Gains. Basically, the Fat Loss Forever approach incorporates a full day of cheating followed by a 36-hour fast. The rest of the week uses the other methods of fasting. This method has a schedule arranged which makes it easier to plan your week accordingly. The structure also helps your body get used to a set schedule so it does not feel like it is suffering on the other days.

Generally, Romaniello and Go recommend performing the 36-hour fast on a day when you are at your busiest. It helps to keep your mind off of food and your impending hunger. Romaniello and Go also include a workout plan to go with the Fat Loss Forever fasting schedule.

The great part of the Fat Loss Forever fasting method is that you do get a cheat day once a week. Unfortunately, if you have a hard time controlling yourself on your cheat days due to restriction, you may undo all of your hard work during your fast. If you are very good at controlling yourself, your cheat days can supplement your diet very well. Also, a 36-hour fasting period may be hard for some people. You may want to keep yourself busy throughout the day or consume a large quantity of water or caffeine to keep the hunger pains at bay.

My favorite way of keeping busy is to fast on a chore day because there is so much to do, but I have never attempted a 36-hour fast so I cannot really say how well that will work. I do know that if I am ever bored with massive amounts of snacks surrounding me, I will never be able to concentrate so I make sure to keep busy if I choose to fast for a large amount of time. Whatever makes it easier, right?

Myths of Intermittent Fasting

Many myths exist in the health and fitness world. Quite a few myths have formed over the years in regards to Intermittent Fasting. How many of them hold any real ground? Let's see if their foundation is more solid than sand!

Intermittent Fasting Slows Metabolism

For years, we have believed that eating 5-6 small meals throughout the day instead of 3 large meals will lead to weight loss. That works mainly if your small meals are indeed small in calories. Scientists and nutritionists had us believing that eating consistently would help increase our metabolism and keep it active, and that prolonging meals when you feel hunger will decrease your metabolism. We have been manipulated into thinking that our bodies will go into starvation mode just because we skip a meal.

Recent studies have disproved that theory. Researchers have found that your metabolism only slows if you fast for periods longer than 60 hours. Hear that? If you do not eat for longer than two and a half days, your metabolism will slow. I am pretty sure you will break down and eat before then, but I just want to let you know, eat before your fast lasts 3 days!

Deficiencies in Nutrients

There are some people who argue that people who practice Intermittent Fasting are less likely to meet their nutrient needs. Yes, everyone should consume a certain amount of nutrients daily. If you fast for a 24-hour period, you may not be able to get those nutrients during your fasting days, but if you consume 500 calories during that day, you can make up those nutrients or consume those necessary nutrients on non-fasting days.

That is not to say that there are not some people who absolutely abuse the system and just consume junk foods because they do fast intermittently. Yes, you can fit that burger from McDonald's, but if you are thinking about your health, you will not actually be consuming pizzas and burgers all day. If you want to feel satisfied, eat your vegetables and fruits. You will definitely get your nutrients that way, do you hear me?

Skipping Breakfast will Lead to Fat Gain

Breakfast is considered the most important meal of the day. Why? In the morning, after you have woken up from your "fast," your blood sugar is at its lowest as well as your blood pressure. Your insulin sensitivity is at its highest after an overnight fast, as well, so it is the most optimal time to eat a meal. If you happen to suffer from low blood pressure in the morning, you will find that eating a meal will help get you back into functionality so that you do not accidentally end up fainting or losing focus on what the day has ahead of you!

There have been studies that have showed that people who skip breakfast lose weight. What they generally do not tell you is that these women tend to be "on-the-go" usually so they usually eat whatever is convenient which can be drive thru foods, fast food, or junk foods from any convenience store. If you eat like that every day, day in and day out, you are sure to gain weight.

However, what happens if you are choosing to skip breakfast and just fast longer?

Well, if you are making the conscious decision to intermittently fast, you already probably know how you will eat the rest of the day or how to make a healthy decision for your weight loss plan. You are not just skipping breakfast out of convenience. If you are putting a lot of thought into your own diet, you will not be gaining weight just because you skip a meal.

Intermittent Fasting is Bad for Women

Some people like to argue that Intermittent Fasting is bad for women. People think that it can negatively affect hormone levels and glucose tolerance as well as lead to decreased satisfaction and frequent hunger in women. While some studies support that theory, other studies have shown that women may continue practicing Intermittent Fasting without any effect on their bodies or hunger levels.

As a woman, I can attest that sometimes, I am just sick of dieting, but that has something to do more with when I was counting macronutrients and my calorie intake than my practicing Intermittent Fasting. I love Intermittent Fasting. I have more control of how much I take into my body and feel like I am able to achieve more satisfaction with my meals if I can intake more due to my fasting throughout the day.

Do I miss eating breakfast? Not really. I miss eating breakfast foods from fast food restaurants, which are bad for you anyway. I can still eat breakfast foods for dinner or lunch if I want. Sure, I cannot get that chorizo biscuit from Carl's Jr that may be bad for my body and daily calorie intake, but I can always make something like it at home for cheaper with fewer calories. I prefer skipping breakfast anyway so that I can train fasted and not worry about packing or making a breakfast before work. Who needs extra work in the morning? That is just time taken away from me playing with my phone or sleeping in!

Fasted Training is Bad for You

There was a time when people thought fasted training was great for burning fat, especially if you -are performing cardio. Professional weightlifters were worried that fasted training can cause catabolism, which is the breaking down of muscle. This is also the reason why some athletes attempt to consume something about 30 minutes after a workout so that they can meet a "metabolic window."

Recent studies have showed that even 60 minutes of running while fasted will insignificantly affect your muscle growth. Fasted training will not negatively affect your strength performance as once was thought.

However, there is still some unease when it comes to fasted weight training due to the ability to synthesize protein. To help aid in the synthesizing of proteins, it is recommended to consume up to 10mg of BCAA (branched chain amino acids) before and after weight training.

Eating Large Meals at Night Will Make You Gain Weight

You may have heard of this saying before: "Eat like a king in the morning, eat like a prince for lunch, and eat like a pauper for dinner." What does that even mean? It basically means eat your smallest meals at night and your biggest meals in the morning. The idea is that consuming large meals at night make you gain a lot of weight.

While, eating large amounts of carbs at night will make you weigh more in the morning than if you were to consume just protein; that is only due to the fact that consuming more carbs means your body will retain more water. More carbs means more water weight. That makes sense, doesn't it? Carbohydrates tend to hold onto more water than proteins or fats.

Recent studies have shown that consuming large meals at night does not make you gain more fat. Actually, recent studies have shown that your meal times do not matter. Have you not eaten throughout the day? Then feel free to eat at night. If you feel like just fasting throughout the day and eating one meal at night, feel free to.

The professional competitive eater, Sonya Thomas, also known as The Black Widow, consumes one large meal at the end of a day instead of small meals throughout the day. You may think that competitive eaters are heavy set individuals, but she will definitely surprise you.

Eating "Bad" Foods will Make You Fat

It seems that in today's society, we are so quick to dismiss foods that are bad for us like chocolate, chips, pizza, or anything fast food related. One of my coworkers always likes to ask if something is fat free, which is a joke of course, but it always gets me wondering how many people truly pay attention to the fat content of a food.

The thing about "bad" foods is that they are generally high in fats and carbohydrates, and low in protein and fiber. "Bad" foods are also labeled as "unclean" usually, but what makes them "unclean." Generally, people like to think of foods with a lot of chemicals in it "unclean" and those same people will eat a lot of vegetables because they are "clean" and will help with weight loss.

The only reasons why I think that clean foods will aid in weight loss is due to the fact that they are high in fiber to help you feel full and satisfied, and they are low in calories because they mainly contain trace carbohydrates and protein. Aside from that, I do not truly believe that they are imperative in helping you lose weight or ensure you gain only lean muscle. Remember that calories in have to be less than calories out? That rule applies here as well!

If you ate a single personal pizza each day, you are bound to lose weight. You might be miserable since you cannot eat as much as you want or stay full for a longer period of time, but in the end, you will lose weight! Who wants to live on a personal pizza a day? That is just plain sad, right? Eat a vegetable. It will help you with the hunger! However, that is not really the point I was trying to make.

I am just saying that even if foods are labelled "bad" or "unclean," they are not going to cause you to gain weight all of a sudden. Have you ever been in an office where a single donut causes each woman to fall into utter despair? I have. I have coworkers who rag on each other for consuming a piece of chocolate. Hello? It is just a piece! Moderation is key! Have that chocolate if you want, but do not binge! Do not eat more than what you wanted to try!

Plus, with the addition on Intermittent Fasting, you can save yourself a great deal of guilty by saving up your calories for later so that you can stay full before bed or eat a nice treat. Do not put so much pressure on yourself for eating something labelled as "unclean!"

Here is a short story. I used to focus on eating clean. I was riddled with guilt if I ever ate something small or did not eat any vegetables in a day. Yeah, that sucks. It is super important to eat vegetables! Usually, when I was going through my orthorexia, I had a very difficult time if the people around me wanted to eat. I felt like my choices were limited to the salads, but I always wanted something else. Who likes to eat salads when they eat out?

I would rather eat a sandwich! Hell, I'd take the steak or fish! Yet, I always felt guilty if I did not eat at least 5 cups of vegetables and fruits a day, or if I ate out. I became irritable. I yelled a lot. I found my sanity slipping for stupid reasons like eating out or a lack of healthy eating options. Is that not sad? I look back now and think about how irrational I was. I felt very bad, but these things do happen.

Since I started Intermittent Fasting and counted my caloric intake properly, I regained a bit of my sanity, but it was when I quit counting calories that I truly felt alive. Do I worry about weight gain? Sometimes, but I know it is not a big deal so these days, I am retaining my sanity. I think that is a great sign. Each day I return little by little to a normal mindset. I can eat out now without feeling like a terrible person. I can get the mozzarella sticks if I want to! I can get a hamburger!

Intermittent Fasting has helped heal my relationship with "unclean" foods and eased the heavy pressure I was placing upon myself to eat a certain way to ensure proper weight loss. Intermittent Fasting combined with flexible dieting has helped restore my sanity so that I can continue to function the same way I did as a child. Do you not miss that childish and naive innocence you had when you were little? Sometimes I do. Life gets hard and society's ideals are an unbearable burden on anyone's shoulders, do you not agree?

Nutrition

A major part of Intermittent Fasting is eating. Yes, that sounds self-explanatory, doesn't it? Let me explain. Eating is very important in our day-to-day lives and we must consider what we consume very carefully. With Intermittent Fasting, you can consume higher calorie foods like that six-dollar burger from Carl's Jr or that pasta from Olive Garden without worrying too much about excessive fat gain, but you do have to ensure that your body gets its proper nutrients.

Even though you are using Intermittent Fasting for some flexible dieting, lower calorie foods with a high nutrition profile will help you feel full longer. It is that fiber that fills your stomach! And well, fiber also gets your system moving, if you know what I mean.

If you are practicing the Alternate Day Diet or the 5:2 diet, you will find that if you consume a burger for your 500 calories, you will starve before you sleep. Yeah, that burger may taste great, but it will not fill your stomach enough. Plus, you will not get to eat the fries! How can you get a burger without fries?

On the days when you need to consume about 500 calories, it is best to consume 500 calories in vegetables because you will fill your stomach up and feel satisfied. I do not know about you, but most of the time, if I eat a small meal before bed, I will not be able to sleep. I need to eat to sleep! It sounds funny but it is true!

Like I mentioned in the previous section, you can still lose weight when you consume "bad" foods, but what is important is that you eat fewer calories than your body burns in a day. Do not let food consume your thoughts. If you want to eat out, go for it, but also make note that you should make healthy choices or eat healthy foods the rest of the day.

Eating junk food all day may sound appealing but the sugar and salt will definitely have you buzzing more than if you had been drinking. Speaking of drinking, try to avoid drinking your calories. Those go by fast and you will miss them when they are!

Sure, you can have a Starbucks Frappuccino, but have you seen how many calories are in one? Or how much sugar is in it? My favorite drink, the caramel ribbon crunch Frappuccino, in a Venti size without whipped cream can be over 60 grams of sugar. Seriously, beware!

Also, it is really important to remember that while alcohol can be great, it can have some negative side effects. Alcohol is an empty calorie drink which means it does not help your body run at all. You are just drinking calories! It does not even become usable energy for your body to use! Another important note to keep in mind is that alcohol does eat muscle.

What does that mean exactly? If you drink alcohol, it can eat away at your muscle and make you actually lose muscle. Is that not sad? You put all that work into gaining some sort of muscle mass, do not ruin it by downing your body weight in alcohol, alright? That is just not a smart move, especially since alcohol does have calories. They do not just burn away as empty calories!

Here is a special tip:

If you are going to work out in the morning or while fasted, consume a cup of coffee or caffeine. A cup of coffee before any exercise routine will increase your metabolism and cause you to burn more when you workout. Plus, it gives you that energy boost you need to keep working hard. Is that not a great tip?

My favorite drink from Starbucks is from the secret menu called "The Black Widow" (not to be confused with the competitive eater) which is just iced black tea and iced black coffee. It will give you a great kick and suppress any appetite you might have until you finish fasting. You are welcome!

Training

People who are devoted to their physical fitness or people who want to lose weight may want to include physical fitness training into their daily schedules. One aspect of physical fitness training involves weight training, which is essential for building a faster metabolism because while the body is at rest, it will burn more if the body contains more muscle. That means you are able to eat more to maintain your body weight! Who does not want that?

If you lift weights that are heavy enough to create some difficulty for you, you can build more muscle and even get your heart pumping. An elevated heart rate means you are burning more!

Here is a little advice for you, just because I care: Do not forget leg day! First of all, the muscles in your legs are amongst the largest in your body. You know that muscle you loved to say as a child? Yes, the gluteus maximus! The gluteus maximus is the largest muscle in the body.

If you do not work it out, you are missing out on training one of the major muscles and you are severely limiting your metabolic potential! Do not handicap yourself by forgetting such a great muscle.

Second of all, have you ever seen those guys at the gym that workout their upper body almost every single day but look a little off kilter? Yeah, well, they forgot leg day. They typically have skinny looking legs that make their bodies so off balance. I have a friend who only works out the muscles he sees so typically his legs and certain parts of his upper body are smaller.

Do not be that guy. Do not forget to evenly train your muscles! Balance is key! It gets a whole lot harder to fix that once you have developed a lot in one area but are underdeveloped in another.

Performing cardio is also essential to weight loss. It can create a large calorie deficit if you put the effort into it, but it is also very good for your heart. Heart health can be maintained by proper cardio. While I do not agree that you should utilize cardio for your weight loss because the amount of dislike people have associated with cardio which will only lead to more distaste for cardio in the future, I do believe that cardiovascular fitness in maintaining proper health so even if your goal is not to lose weight, I think it is important to continue performing cardio, but in moderate quantities. Do not make yourself hate cardio by forcing yourself through long episodes of cardio workouts, which I know all too well.

Studies have gone back and forth on many aspects of physical fitness and weight loss, but if you want to optimize your fat loss, perform your cardio after your weight training. If you perform your weight training after your cardio workouts, you may find you have expended most of your energy so you cannot properly perform as well as you could have. Although it is important to warm up your muscles, do not tire them out with a long cardio workout.

Aside from optimizing your workouts, if you do perform your cardio workouts after your weight lifting workouts, your body has been proven to burn more fat than if you were to reverse the order of your workout, so if the idea did not entice you at first, at least you can look forward to burning more fat with this workout routine! Think of that as a secret workout life hack! You are welcome!

Of course, your body does require a certain amount of calories to properly operate. If you are at a constant caloric deficit while weight training, all you can attempt to do is keep the amount of muscle you have. You will not be gaining any muscle through a caloric deficit, so if you are trying to lose weight, you will find at the end of your weight loss period, your body will gain weight on the same amount of calories you were consuming before when you were maintaining your weight. It is a very sad fact of dieting.

An important note to take is that you should not be training extraneously when fasted. That is not to say that you cannot workout when you are fasting. Studies have gone back and forth regarding fat loss with fasted workouts. Like I said earlier, all that matters is if the calories you expend is more than the calories you intake. If your body does not perform well starved, do not work out fasted! It works for some but not all. If you do train fasted, though, you should make sure to eat a proper meal sometime after you train.

Make sure that your meal is balanced so you have protein or muscle repair and carbohydrates for energy. While I do not truly believe that your muscles can become "catabolic," it is important to eat to restore your energy. I hate when I feel completely fatigued the rest of the day after working out!

I did state earlier that I do train early mornings before work, but still continue to fast after. I have not noticed a large amount of muscle loss at all unless my intake decreases drastically. I prefer to work out in the mornings because the gym is less crowded, I can just get my workout out of the way and go on with my life. Also, statistics show that if you schedule your workouts in the morning, you will most likely perform them compared to if your workouts are in the evenings, which, through experience, I can attest to.

Anyway, I fast until later in the day to prevent myself from binge eating. Training fasted also makes my cardio sessions easier since there is nothing to hinder me or make me feel lethargic. This was mainly through trial and error, but that is how my body responds. Like I have expressed often throughout this article, you should do what works best for your body! All of our bodies do not function or react the same!

With that in mind, you must tailor your workouts according to how your body reacts. Some people develop certain body parts a lot faster. For me, my calves develop fairly quickly, which I can tell by the immense pain in my shins when I run. Some people's glutes may grow faster, but some people may not grow muscle easily at all.

This does not just apply for muscles. Some bodies just burn fat faster and not gain any easily, while others gain fat quickly and cannot even get the fat off. It just is not fair, is it? You just need to figure out what type of body you have and figure out what types of workouts work best for you. We may not be all gifted genetically, but that does not mean we cannot do anything about it!

Let Us Get Started!

Now that you have all of this information, where do you start? Most people will research how to lose weight, but most of the time, no one actually utilizes that knowledge. First off, which Intermittent Fasting schedule suits your personality and schedule? Do you think you have the willpower to fast through a whole day or maybe you just want to fast for a short period of time so you can eat more every day.

Did you pick what type of fasting schedule would suit your needs? Now you have to figure out when you will fast. Do you want to fast right after dinner so you can eat an early lunch if you would like? Do you want to fast right after dinner until dinner tomorrow? Or maybe you would prefer if you could fast until dinner 2 days later. Just make sure that the fasting day you schedule is on a busy day. Keep it busy, guys!

Counting calories is always an option, even though you are fasting. It makes the math work out so much better, but it can be a great hassle. If you do not count calories, you can still create a meal plan and make sure that your meals are full of healthy ingredients. Prepping your meals makes it a lot easier to stay on track so you may want to pack your meals on your fasting days as a way to keep busy.

Lastly, you just have to think about proper training. You should plan your training days on a different day from your fasting days. You need the calories to feed your body and have energy to actually exercise! Who wants to drop a barbell when their squatting? That is just dangerous! I know I hate looking like a weakling when I have to drop to a lower weight just because I feel weak.

Planning a proper exercise routine seems like a daunting task at first. I put more thought into my workout routine than what I eat to be honest. I want to hit every muscle at least twice a week if possible! I do not want my muscles to detrain. I put way too much work into my body to let it derail itself just because I train each muscle group once a week.

Mr. Olympia, Phil Heath, has stated that he makes sure to hit each muscle group twice a week to prevent the muscles from detraining. I am not saying you are going to suddenly look like Phil Heath—that will not happen no matter how much you might fear it will—but if the strongest man in the world says he trains twice a week to build muscle, why should we not at least consider his advice?

If you split your workout routine into lower body and upper body, you can hope to hit each muscle group three times in a week, but that means you would spend a great deal more time doing your upper body than your lower body. A traditional split would be legs, triceps and chest, and then back and biceps. With this routine, you can hit each muscle group twice with a day for rest, which is essential to your body's growth and recovery.

Speaking of which, rest days are crucial for your body to properly recover. It is very tempting to skip them so that you can burn more, but studies have shown that your body reacts better with a rest day. If it bothers you to be so inactive, make it an active rest day so you can go on a hike or a bike ride, but an inactive rest day is much better for your body. Remember to take care of your body!

Who Should Not Do Intermittent Fasting?

Throughout this entire article, I have been preaching that you should do what your body wants. Never do something that will be counterintuitive to what your body wants or how it reacts. If your knees are shaking from hitting the squat rack, do not just add an extra 50 pounds! What type of logic is that? This same thinking is crucial when it comes to Intermittent Fasting.

Who exactly should not practice Intermittent Fasting? Earlier, I did state that those who suffer from acid reflux should avoid it, but who else should not do Intermittent Fasting? Well, if you happen to be diabetic, Intermittent Fasting may cause some issues by causing risk associated with low blood glucose levels unless you are willing to make some arrangements beforehand to prevent any complications in the future due to fasting.

Generally any woman who is pregnant should speak with a physician prior to making any dire changes in her daily life, but the same advice can be given to any individual, especially when it revolves around proper diet and nutrition. Also, people who suffer from anemia or take certain medications should think twice before attempting anything like Intermittent Fasting.

You have to remember that if you do not feel well when you skip breakfast for even a few hours, you should not try to practice

Intermittent Fasting, although I do know some individuals who start fasting late in the afternoon so they can break their fast in the morning the next day. If that happens to work for you, then try it.

As for me, I do have some lethargy on some days or lightheadedness on other days, but for the most part, I may not even notice that I have not eaten breakfast yet. This is especially true when I keep busy by working or doing chores. If I have slow days or free time, I tend to think about food, but I manage to keep my fasting windows for the most part. Sometimes, however, I do lack self-control so when I finally break my fast, I may indulge a great deal and there are times when I am prone to binging.

I do not know what triggers it, but to prevent it, I avoid buying any small snacks I know I will snack excessively on like pretzels, nuts, and of course, chips! Chips are infamous for being a major binge food. I never feel full snacking on them and they disappear so quickly! Is it not a travesty? Knowing how your brain works also helps when it comes to self-control. Do not let yourself have any easy access to certain foods that you may not be able to control yourself around.

So There You Have It – Intermittent Fasting!

I hope that you got a lot of information in this book. There is a lot to think about, isn't there? Intermittent Fasting is a very handy method of dieting or eating so that you can have some flexibility in your eating and improve your health.

If you think you are interested in transitioning to Intermittent Fasting, take it slow and steady. The most important part of your health, regardless of lean muscle gain or weight loss, is to listen to your body. No matter what path you take, do what is best for your health. Remember, weight loss can be stressful so take on as much stress as you think can handle because we are all warriors!

Intermittent Fasting is all about flexibility and making dieting easier. It will take away some of the stress and make your attempts at losing weight simpler. Calorie counting may work for some, but a lot of us just cannot waste our time with it. I am not going to say that Intermittent Fasting is the "cure for all" weight loss technique, but can truly transform how we deal with weight loss and lean muscle gain.

Dealing with your weight is a pain, but it does not have to be impossible. Make it easier by trying new methods and finding out what works for you. Try Intermittent Fasting. It changed my life. I feel more at ease and more confident that I am taking the right actions for myself.

Now, what do you think is right for you?

*****

If you've enjoyed this book, **please** consider leaving a review and letting others know what you thought!